Prof. Dr. Luis E. Abad Pedraza

MANUAL FOR OPHTHALMOLOGY TECHNICATURE

Imprint
Any brand names and product names mentioned in this book are subject to trademark, brand or patent protection and are trademarks or registered trademarks of their respective holders. The use of brand names, product names, common names, trade names, product descriptions etc. even without a particular marking in this work is in no way to be construed to mean that such names may be regarded as unrestricted in respect of trademark and brand protection legislation and could thus be used by anyone.

Cover image: www.ingimage.com

This book is a translation from the original published under ISBN 978-3-659-70159-7.

Publisher:
Sciencia Scripts
is a trademark of
Dodo Books Indian Ocean Ltd. and OmniScriptum S.R.L publishing group

120 High Road, East Finchley, London, N2 9ED, United Kingdom
Str. Armeneasca 28/1, office 1, Chisinau MD-2012, Republic of Moldova, Europe
Printed at: see last page
ISBN: 978-620-6-06867-9

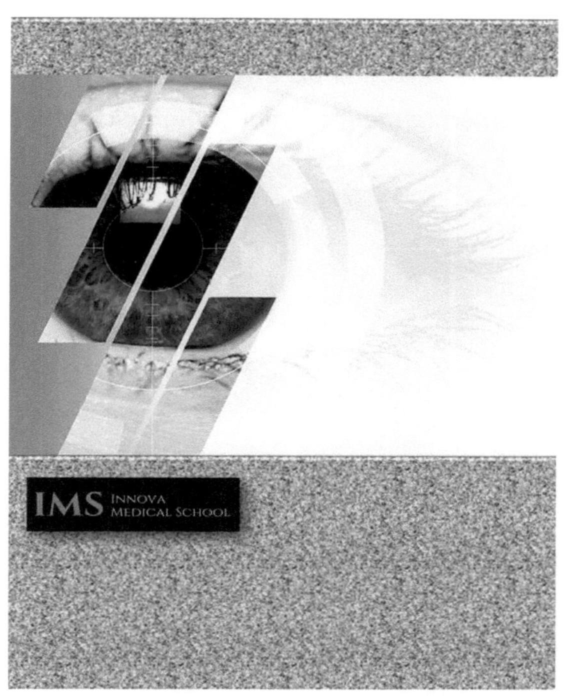

OPHTHALMOLOGY TECHNICIAN

OPHTHALMOLOGY TECHNICIAN

SECOND PART "BASIC UNDERSTANDING OF OPHTHALMOLOGIC PATHOLOGY".

PROF. DR. LUIS E. ABAD PEDRAZA

Ophthalmology Technician

Part Two

"Basic understanding of ophthalmologic pathology"

DEDICATION

To my wife, Silvana, for accompanying me on all my specialization trips and giving me her unconditional help, and to my sons Danilo and Marcos for filling me with love and enthusiasm to continue in this task.

Prof. Dr. Luis E. Abad Pedraza

FOREWORD

This book aims, through scientific knowledge, to present in an easy, concise and basic way, the most frequent diseases that cause changes in different ocular structures, some of them triggering severe alterations of vision, and even blindness.I am confident that this study manual will allow a better evaluation, making a more appropriate analysis, helping to have a better understanding of the problem. With this brief introduction, I would like to make this work available to you, hoping that it will be a means for all of us to improve the quality of technical collaboration in Ophthalmology, for the benefit of the patient and thus achieve our intention.

Kind regards,

Prof. Dr. Luis E. Abad Pedraza

INDEX

INTRODUCTION

"Better is the health that was never lost."

Seneca

Health is one of the components of community development and is directly related to the availability and distribution of resources. The health promoter is a promoter of healthy habits, we understand by health promotion activities, those that are carried out to reinforce healthy habits and to prevent risk factors. He/she is an indispensable agent in the territory for the prevention of disease and to favor the population's access to health.The purpose of this manual is to provide knowledge about visual pathologies in order to promote prevention, early detection and timely referral for treatment.In view of the importance of contributing to the knowledge of health agents (technicians and auxiliaries), the aim is to increase the number of human resources and technicians in the regions that need them, in order to avoid secondary complications through training. The aim is to provide knowledge to human resources in order to develop screening tasks and early referral of pathologies of the visual field and to implement health promotion lines.

CHAPTER 1

THE EYE

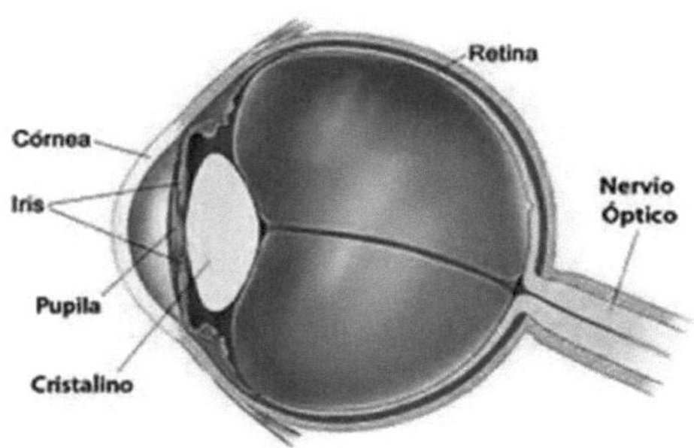

The eyeball, through its structures, receives external luminous stimuli, encodes them and transmits them through the optical pathway to the brain, where the phenomenon of vision occurs.

ANATOMY OF THE EYE

The eye is spheroidal in shape and consists of three concentric layers:

1. **Outer tunic:** cornea and sclera.
2. **Middle or vascular tunic:** uvea, formed by iris, ciliary body and choroid.
3. **Inner tunic:** retina.

In its interior there are limited compartments:

1. **Anterior chamber**, bounded by the posterior aspect of the cornea in front, and the iridopupillary diaphragm behind. It is occupied by aqueous humor.
2. **Posterior chamber**, between the iris and pupil anteriorly and the anterior aspect of the lens, with its zonular fibers. Occupied by aqueous humor.

3. **Vitreous chamber**, limited by the posterior face of the crystalline lens, posterior fibers of the zonule and part of the ciliary body in front and the rest by the retina. It is occupied by the vitreous.

Cornea

A transparent structure that provides much of the refractive power necessary to focus light on the retina. It also functions as a protective structure for intraocular tissues and humors. The cornea has abundant sensory innervation. It is characterized by being avascular and transparent.

Sclera

A fibrous membrane of whitish appearance, very resistant, that protects the intraocular tissues. Its posterior portion is perforated by the optic nerve and by the entrance and exit of blood vessels. The episclera is a lax vascularized tissue that covers the sclera and reacts strongly to inflammation of the sclera.

Iris

A colored membrane, perforated in its center by a circular hole, the pupil. Its function is to limit the light entering the eye.

and the accessory glands. The main gland is located under the superoexternal angle of the orbit, the rest of the accessory glands are located in: tarsal conjunctiva, bulbar, conjunctival sac fundus and in the conjunctiva of the palpebral free edge. Tears form a tear film that forms a barrier between the corneal-conjunctival epithelium and the external environment. Their role is defense against infections, corneal nutrition and optical perfection of the air-cornea diopter.A deficient secretion will give a dry eye syndrome, a deficient evacuation will result in lacrimation or epiphora. The lacrimal ducts are located in the inferointernal region of the orbit. They start at the lacrimal puncta, one superior and one inferior. These points continue with the lacrimal canaliculi that converge in a common canaliculus, which continues with the lacrimal sac. Its lower end continues with the lacrimonasal canal that flows into the inferior meatus of the nose.

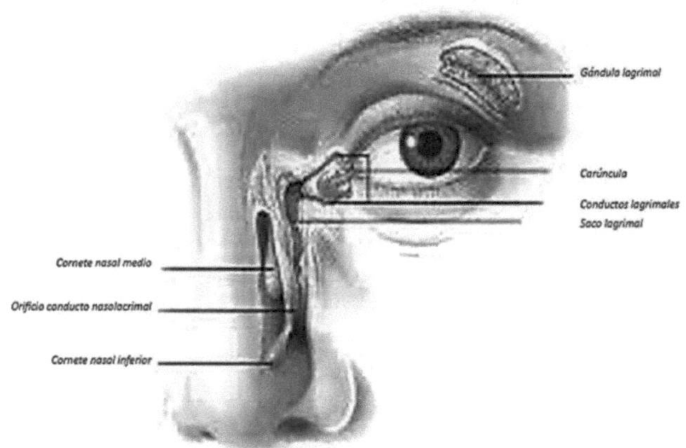

Eye Functioning

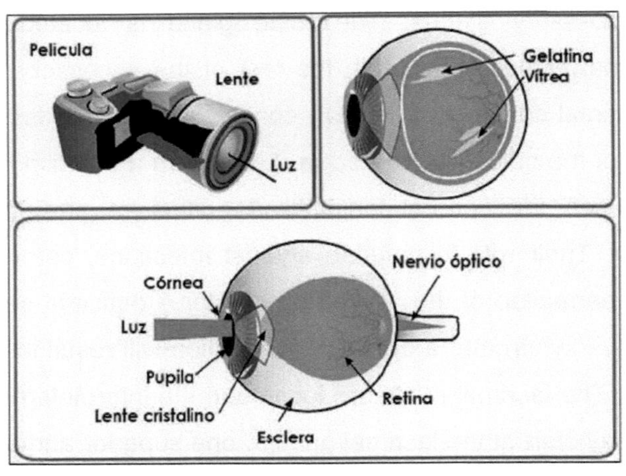
Pelicula
Lente
Luz
Gelatina
Vítrea
Nervio óptico
Córnea
Luz
Pupila
Lente cristalino
Esclera
Retina

CHAPTER 2
VISUAL ACUITY

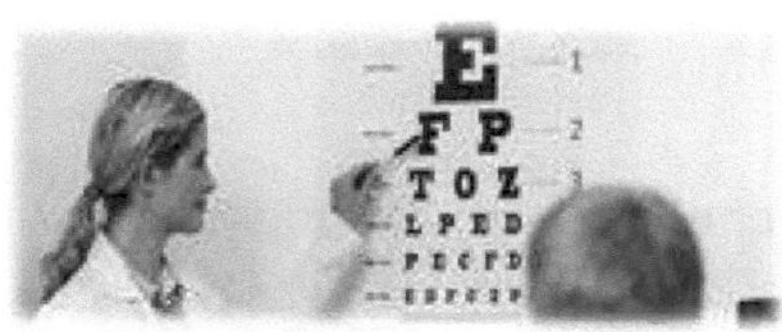

The acuity is I ability of the system division system to perceive, detect Identify objector a given distance.

VISUAL ACUITY

Visual acuity is the ability of the vision system to perceive, detect or identify objects at a given distance. It indicates the **quality of vision**. It depends on the anatomo-functional integrity of the visual apparatus (transparency of the ocular media - cornea, crystalline lens, aqueous humor and vitreous - and retinal functionality).

CONSTITUTES A MANDATORY EXAMINATION, WHICH GIVES US GLOBAL INFORMATION ON THE FUNCTIONALITY OF THE VISUAL SYSTEM.

Visual acuity is quantified through the Optotypes sign, which can be signs, letters, numbers or drawings of decreasing sizes, at a certain distance. Far: 3 mts.

We can evaluate visual acuity:

- Without optical correction (without glasses)
- Optically corrected (with glasses)

This will depend on whether the patient has glasses or not, and in case he/she has them, we must always evaluate him/her both ways (with and without correction).

Visual Acuity Test

Technique to evaluate visual acuity

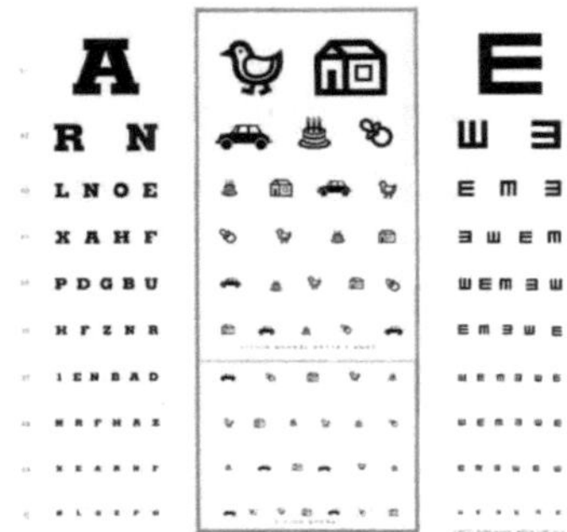

1- Ensure good illumination of the environment and if possible good illumination of the optotypes.

2- Place the patient 3 meters away from the sign.

3- Take the VA of each eye separately, instructing the patient to occlude first one eye and then the other with the palm of his or her hand.

4- In case the patient has glasses, take the VA of each eye without their lenses and then with their lenses covering one eye and then the other, occluding with, for example, a paper folded in a triangular shape.

5- The VA value corresponds to the smallest row that the patient can read.

Visual acuity is expressed as a fraction, and depends on the number of lines on the poster that the patient can see clearly.The sign will have 10 lines, of different sizes, which will be placed from top to bottom, from the largest to the smallest.

Therefore, the VA may be, for example:

- 1/10: pac that sees only the largest line.

- 4!10: pac. See the 4 largest lines.

- 10/10, in case the patient sees all 10 lines of the poster.

THE NORMAL VISUAL ACCURACY OF AN ADULT PATIENT IS 10/10 or 20/20

Near vision can usually be altered in patients over 40 years old, because presbyopia begins at that age. Presbyopia is an age-related condition, the patient over 40 years old begins to have difficulty seeing near objects, to solve it, patients should use near correction.

Therefore, it is very important to keep in mind that patients over 40 years of age may have difficulty seeing far, near, or both.

Patients will always be referred to an ophthalmologist if they have:

- visual acuity less than 10/10 with or without correction
- difficulty seeing up close

Visual acuity in children

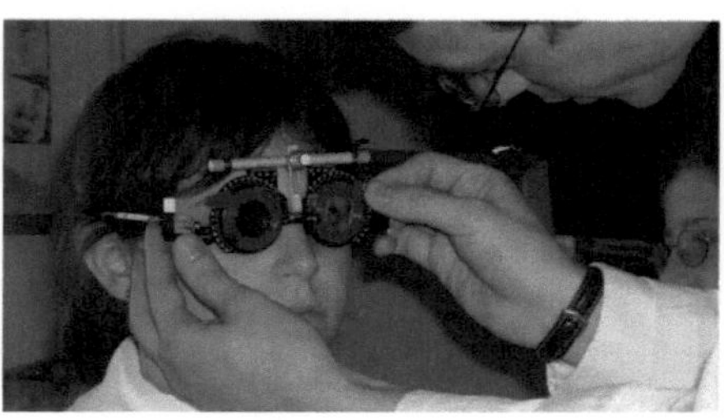

The method to be used for evaluation depends on the age of the child. To determine it, each eye should always be evaluated separately. Two lines of difference between the eyes will be sufficient reason for referral. Visual acuity can be assessed with optotypes from the age of 3 years. In children who do not yet know the letters, it will be evaluated with the letters E.In school children, visual acuity will be evaluated with the Snellen Chart. The student stands 3 meters away from the poster or sheet with the Snellen Optotypes, with good light (preferably located behind the observer) and occludes (covers) one and the other eye for selective assessment of vision. It is suggested that occlusion be performed with the palm of the hand cupped; do not put too much pressure on the occluded eye. It is beneficial for the systematics of the examination to instruct the child to always occlude the right eye first; in this way, the results will always be dumped in the same way: Right Eye / Left Eye.

VISUAL ACUITY VARIES WITH AGE AND AFTER THE AGE OF FIVE, CHILDREN REACH 8/10 TO 10/10 VISION.

That is to say: out of ten lines, 8 should be seen correctly. With a lower vision, a referral to a specialist should be made and also if there are differences of more than 2 lines between eye and eye.

Decimal	Fracción	Snellen (6 m)	Snellen (20 pies)	logMAR
0,10	1/10	6/60	20/200	1,0
0,12	1/8	6/48	20/160	0,9
0,16	4/25	6/37,5	20/125	0,8
0,20	1/5	6/30	20/100	0,7
0,25	1/4	6/24	20/80	0,6
0,32	1/3	6/19	20/63	0,5
0,40	2/5	6/15	20/50	0,4
0,50	1/2	6/12	20/40	0,3
0,63	2/3,2	6/9,5	20/32	0,2
0,80	4/5	6/7,5	20/25	0,1
1,00	**1/1**	**6/6**	**20/20**	**0,0**
1,25	5/4	6/4,8	20/16	-0,1

Comparative table of the different interpretations for visual acuity grading.

Amblyopia

By definition it means vague vision (lazy eye), due to the lack of consolidation of visual acuity or the presence of inadequate or insufficient stimuli during the critical period of visual development (before the age of 6 years, depending on the case).

It is the most frequent cause of low visual acuity in children and young adults.

It is 10 times more frequent than any ocular pathology and affects 4% of the population. In most cases they can recover if they receive treatment before the end of the critical period of visual development. The great majority of cases occur due to refractive defects and if treated in time they have a solution. If they do not receive timely treatment they will NOT have the possibility of seeing in the future.

Strabismus

It is the misalignment of the eyes or lack of parallelism of the ocular axes. They are studied and after a thorough analysis we can classify them.

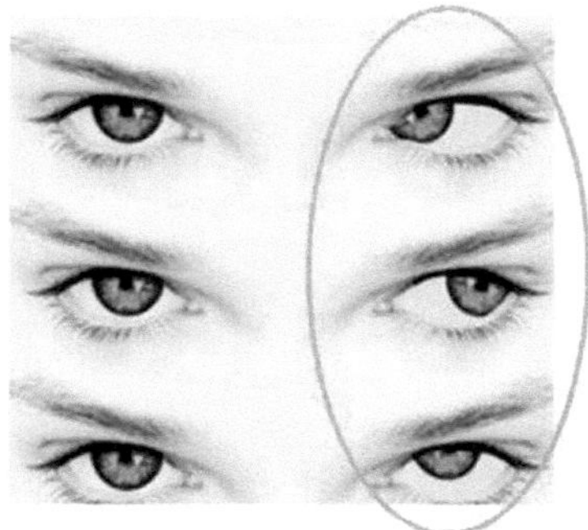

Representation of the different types of ocular deviation.

TENER EN CUENTA QUE LA MAYORÍA DE LAS CAUSAS PUEDEN SER TRATADAS CON ÉXITO EN LA PRIMERA INFANCIA PASADO ESTE PERÍODO NO HAY TRATAMIENTO.CUANTO MÁS PRECOZ ES EL INICIO DEL TRATAMIENTO MEJOR SERÁN LOS RESULTADOS.

CHAPTER 3

OPHTHALMOLOGIC PATHOLOGY

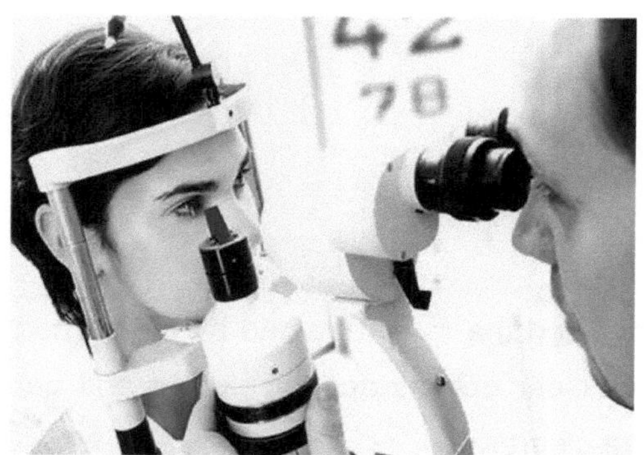

Here we will present the most frequent visual diseases to facilitate their detection and early referral for treatment. This will be determined solely by the ophthalmologist.

REFRACTIVE ERRORS

Myopia

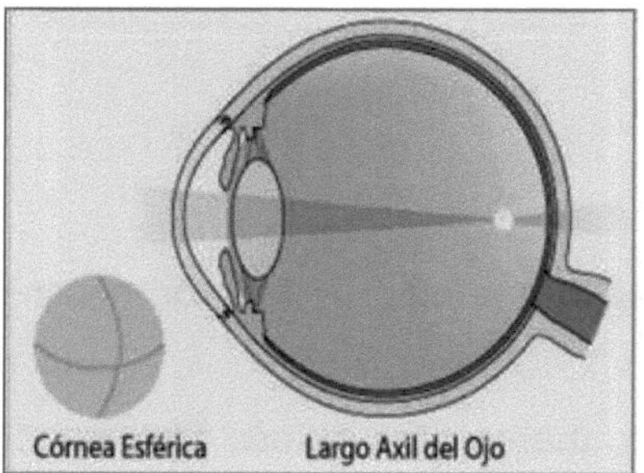

The eye is longer than normal and the rays refracted by the cornea and lens focus in front of the retina. Near objects are seen clearly, but distant objects are blurred.

Hyperopia

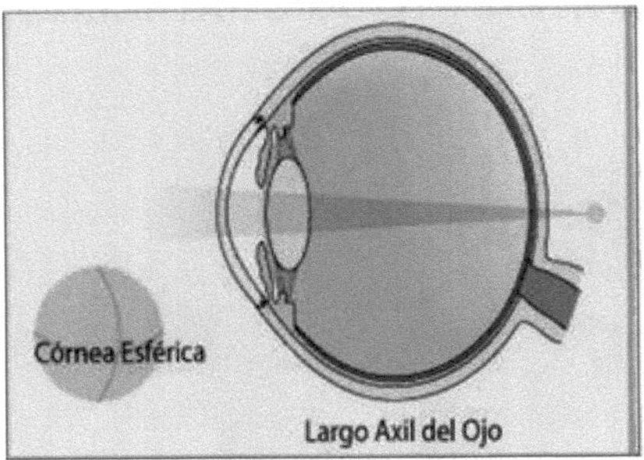

The eye is shorter and the rays refracted by the cornea and lens focus behind the retina. Near objects appear blurred and out of focus, while distant objects are clearer.

Astigmatism

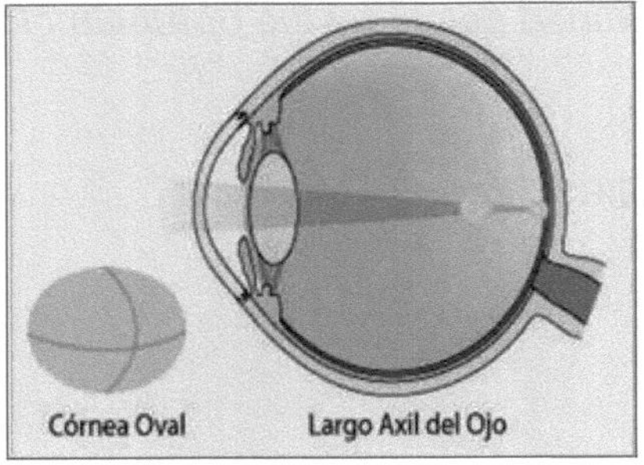

In astigmatism, the rays refracted by the cornea and the crystalline lens focus in two points, therefore instead of a single focus, as occurs in myopia or hyperopia, there are two foci. These foci may be located in front of or behind the retina. This is because the cornea has two radii of curvature, one more curved and the other flatter, similar to a rugby ball.

Presbyopia

When a person is young, the lens is elastic and changes its shape easily, focusing on near and far objects. After the age of 40, it becomes more rigid. Because the lens cannot change its shape as easily as it used to, it becomes more difficult to read up close. This perfectly normal condition is called presbyopia.

CORNEA AND SCLERA

Dry eye

Dry eye is a disease caused by an alteration of tear secretion. Its symptoms are:

- Ocular dryness
- Redness
- Itching
- Ardor
- Grit or foreign body sensation inside the eye
- Tearing
- Ocular fatigue
- Continuous or fluctuating decrease in vision

Adequate lubrication of the eye is possible through a tear balance consisting of good quality tear production and normal blinking. When this balance is broken, or altered by external factors, tear production alters its composition or decreases and there is a possibility of developing dry eye and its consequences. The treatment consists of the administration of artificial tears that act by replacing real tears, that is to say, they soften, protect and lubricate the eyes, allowing the patient to significantly improve his symptoms.

Pterygium

It is a lesion that starts on the ocular conjunctiva and progresses to the cornea.It is more frequent in people who spend a lot of time outdoors, especially during the summer. Prolonged exposure to sunlight, especially ultraviolet rays, and chronic eye irritation due to dry environmental conditions and dust appear to play an important role.

A dry eye can contribute to the development of pterygium. The most common symptoms are:

- Burning sensation
- Itching
- Dryness in the affected eye.

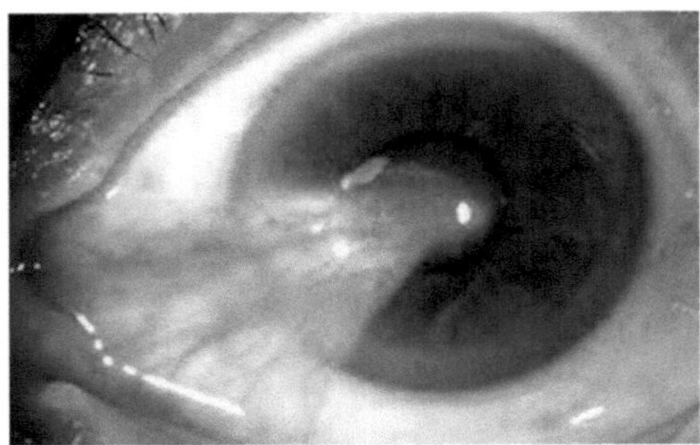

It may reach the point where the pterygium grows large enough to approach the center of the cornea and block the passage of light, producing a marked decrease in vision. In these cases the patient will require surgery to remove the lesion.

Optic nerve

Glaucoma

Glaucoma is a disease of the optic nerve, characterized by a progressive atrophy of the optic nerve due to an increase in ocular pressure. Normal ocular pressure in adults is between 15 and 20 mm Hg and is not related to blood pressure. It can be classified into:

• **Acute:** Acute glaucoma is a pathology in which there is an abrupt and very important increase in eye pressure, usually accompanied by redness of the eye, intense eye and head pain, and sometimes even nausea and vomiting.The most important thing is the rapid treatment to lower the eye pressure.

• **Chronic:** Chronic simple glaucoma or chronic open-angle glaucoma is a chronic disease that affects the optic nerve, which carries vision from the eye to the brain. Therefore, optic nerve involvement results in progressive and irreversible vision loss.

• **Neovascular:** It is a consequence of trobosis or diabetic retinopathy.

The diagnosis of this pathology is based on:

• Ocular pressure measurement

• Optic nerve observation

• Visual field evaluation

In pathology, the increase in ocular pressure generates alteration of the optic nerve (increases its excavation) and consequently alters the visual field. The damages generated are IRREVERSIBLE. Treatment: The objective of the treatment is based on the reduction of ocular pressure, in order to stop the evolution of the disease and prevent damage. Treatment consists in the administration of hypotensive eye drops. If with maximum topical treatment the pressure remains elevated, treatment with argon laser (trabeculoplasty) or laser iridectomy (yag laser), or surgical treatment (trabeculectomy with or without valve placement) will be considered.

CRISTALINO

Waterfall

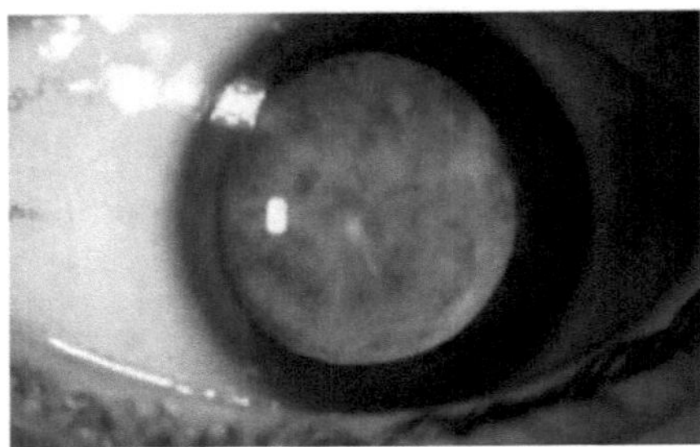

It is a clouding of the lens (crystalline lens) of the eye, which is normally clear and transparent; it can be compared to a window that is frosted with ice or fogged with steam. There are many misconceptions about cataracts.

A waterfall:

- It is not a cloth or layer that covers the eye.
- It is not caused by overuse of the eyes.
- It is not transmitted from one eye to the other.
- It does not cause irreversible blindness.

The common symptoms of cataracts are:

- Vision becomes blurred without pain.

• Glare or sensitivity to light.

• Double vision in one eye.

• Frequent changes in eyeglass prescription.

• Need for more intense light for reading.

• Very poor night vision.

• Colors appear faded or yellowish.

Treatment: surgical, consists in the replacement of the crystalline lens by an intraocular lens.

RETINA

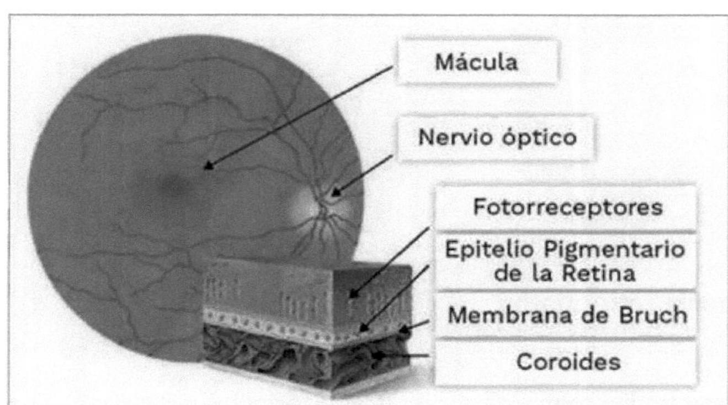

Diabetic retinopathy

Diabetic retinopathy is a complication of diabetes; it is caused by the deterioration of the arteries and veins that irrigate the retina and carry the oxygen and nutrients it needs. This deterioration determines, on the one hand, that liquid can leak out of the vessels, producing edema or swelling of the retina, which prevents it from being able to process images correctly. On the other hand, a shortage of oxygen, also called retinal ischemia, may occur. This ischemia causes the eye, in an attempt to bring more oxygen to the retina, to form new blood vessels, or neovessels, which are fragile and bleed easily. The risks of developing diabetic retinopathy increase as the disease progresses, and depend largely on blood glucose control. Up to 80% of diabetics develop some degree of retinopathy after 15 years of disease progression.

Patients should have their eyes checked annually.

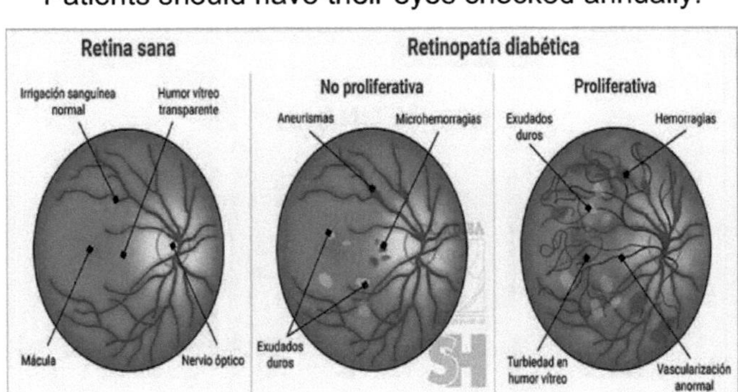

Hypertensive retinopathy

It is damage to the retina as a result of arterial hypertension. The retina is the layer of tissue at the back of the eye that transforms light and images entering the eye into nerve signals that are sent to the brain. High blood pressure can cause damage to the blood vessels in the retina. The higher the blood pressure and the longer it has been elevated, the more likely it is that the damage will be severe.

WHEN THE PATIENT IN ADDITION TO HTA HAS DIABETES, HIGH CHOLESTEROL LEVELS OR SMOKES, HE/SHE PRESENTS A HIGHER RISK OF VISION DAMAGE AND LOSS.

Complications:

• Ischemic optic neuropathy: damage to the nerves in the eye due to poor circulation.

• Retinal artery occlusion: blockage of blood supply to the retinal arteries.

• Retinal vein occlusion

Most people with hypertensive retinopathy have no symptoms until the disease is advanced.

Through the fundus, the doctor can see narrowing of the blood vessels and signs that fluid has leaked from them.

The degree of retinal damage (retinopathy) is graded on a scale of 1 to 4:

• In grade 1, you may have no symptoms.

• Between grades 1 and 4, there are many changes in the blood vessels, areas where blood vessels have leaked, and other parts of the retina.

• Grade 4 hypertensive retinopathy includes edema of the optic nerve and the visual center of the retina (macula). This may cause decreased vision.

The only treatment for hypertensive retinopathy is control of high blood pressure (hypertension).

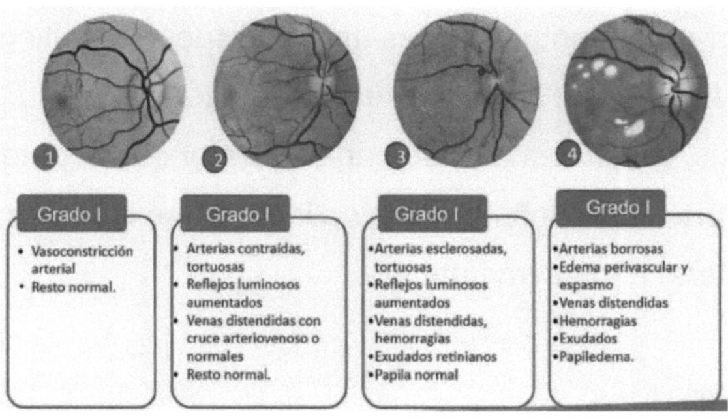

Venous thrombosis

It is the consequence of retinal vein occlusion. It may affect a venous branch or the central retinal vein. When the passage through the vein is closed and as blood continues to enter the tissues through the arteries, venous ingurgitation and subsequent rupture of the capillaries in the territory dependent on that vein occurs due to increased blood pressure retrograde to the point of obstruction.These vascular changes cause a typical image of intraretinal hemorrhages in the affected territory. The clinical picture is usually characterized by an abrupt and painless loss of vision, the amount and significance of which will depend on the retinal territory affected.

Central retinal artery occlusion

This pathology is caused by the obstruction of the central retinal artery. It causes los abrupt of the vision. The cause most frequent causeis arteriosclerosis.

Retinopathy of prematurity

Retinopathy of prematurity (ROP) is an eye disease resulting from immaturity of the retina.This is caused by an alteration in vasculogenesis, which can produce an abnormal development of the same, not all premature infants develop it but when it occurs it is generally bilateral and asymmetrical.

Population to control

• All newborns born preterm - 32 weeks GA (gestational age) and/or less than 1,500 gm BW (birth weight).

•All preterm newborns, over 1500gr. PN and/or 32 weeks' GA who have received oxygen for more than 72 hours or present any of the risk factors.

Frequently associated risk factors are:

• Transfusion with adult hemoglobin;
• Hyperoxia-hypoxia; Acidosis
• Shock. Hypo perfusion; Apneas; Sepsis.
• Resuscitation maneuvers.

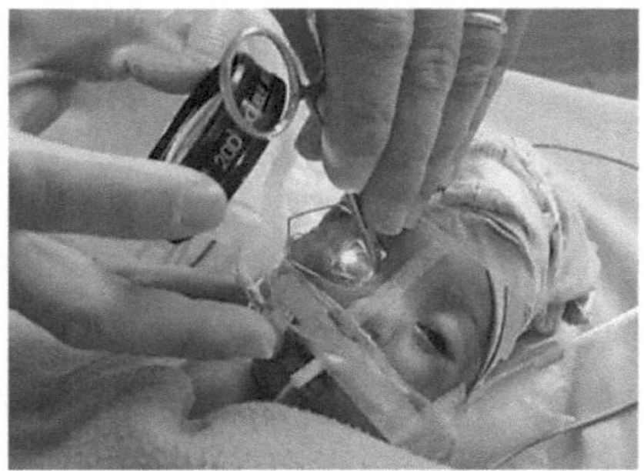

CAMERA

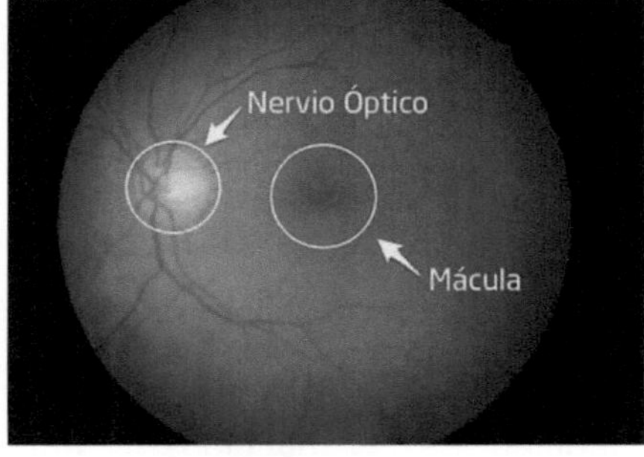

Normal

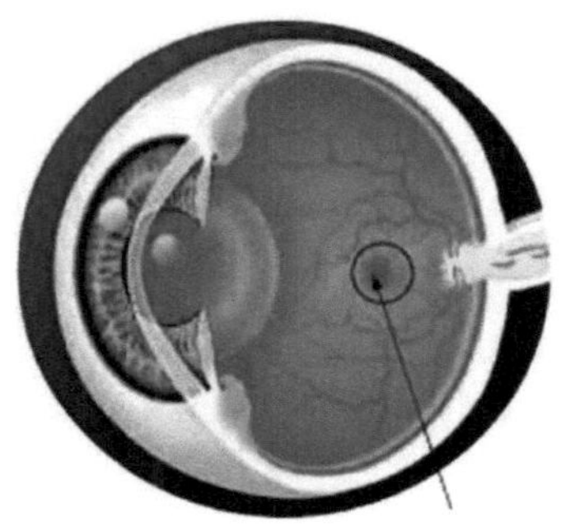

Anatomical location of the macula.

Maculopathy or age-related (or age-associated) macular degeneration (AMD or AMD)

Maculopathy is a condition that compromises central vision, due to alterations that occur in the macula, the part of the retina that makes it possible to read or perceive details in people's faces; age-related maculopathy does not cause pain.In some cases, age-related maculopathy progresses so slowly that people do not notice any change in their vision. In other cases, it progresses more rapidly and can cause vision loss in both eyes. Age-related maculopathy is one of the leading causes of vision loss in people over the age of 60. There are two types:

Dry age-related maculopathy

In dry age-related maculopathy, changes occur in the anatomy of the macula due to the accumulation of yellowish deposits of various sizes called drusen, which cause a progressive deterioration of central vision, which is gradually affected. As dry maculopathy worsens, patients may notice a blurred spot in the center of vision.

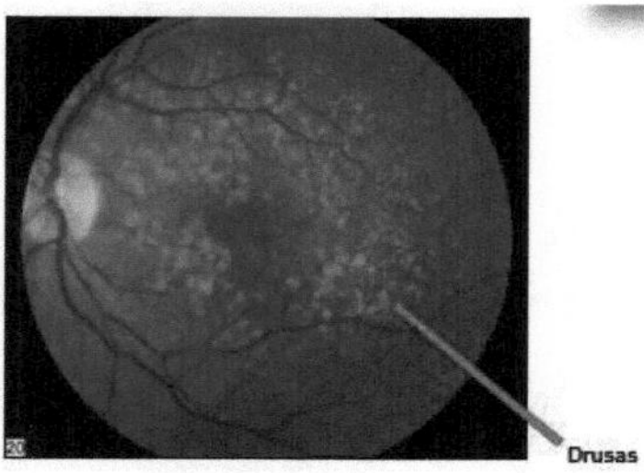

Wet-age-related maculopathy

As a progression of the dry form, the wet form may present, which is characterized by the development of new blood vessels that are abnormal and cause extravasation of fluid, edema and in some cases hemorrhages, which may be related to the development of membranes.

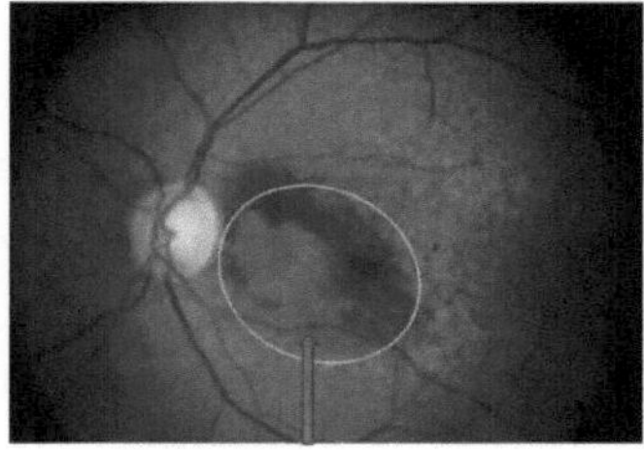

Neovascular membrane

Treatment: Once dry maculopathy reaches the advanced stage, no treatment can prevent vision loss. However, treatment can delay and possibly prevent intermediate maculopathy from progressing to the advanced stage where vision loss occurs. Treatment with antioxidants and zinc is currently available. Wet age-related maculopathy can be treated primarily with antiangiogenic therapy. However, the treatment is by no means curative but aims to reduce or eliminate the adverse effects of the exudation at the macular level.

PARPADOS

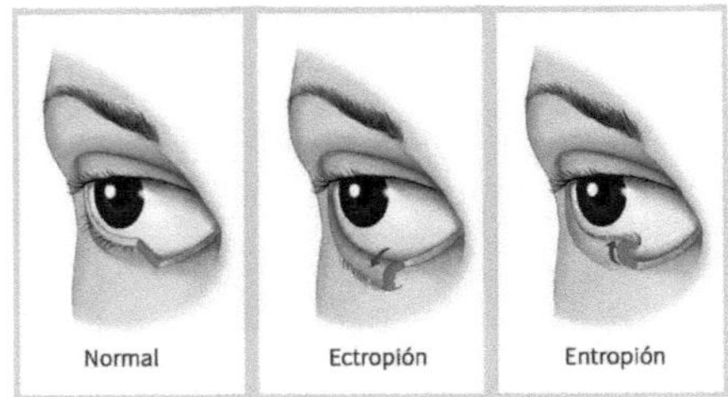

Entropion

It is when the palpebral margin is inverted towards the eyeball. The skin of the palpebral margin and eyelashes rub against the cornea and conjunctiva causing irritation and redness.

Ectropion

The palpebral margin is rotated and inverted with respect to the eyeball.
- MAY CAUSE IRRITATION AND TEARING - MAY CAUSE IRRITATION AND TEARING - MAY CAUSE IRRITATION AND TEARING

Ptosis

Palpebral ptosis (drooping eyelids) is a drooping of the upper eyelid that occludes the eyeball to a variable extent.
The treatment of these pathologies is surgical.

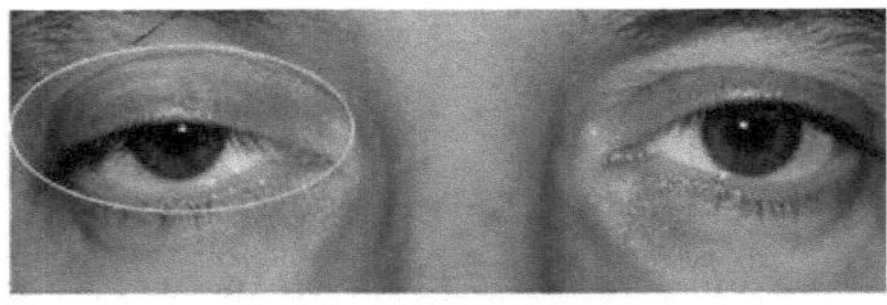

Palpebral ptosis.

Blepharitis

It is the inflammation of the edges of the eyelids, due to inflammation or infection of the Meibomian or Zeiss glands.Seborrheic changes or dandruff are observed on the palpebral margin. It may be a chronic disorder very difficult to eradicate.

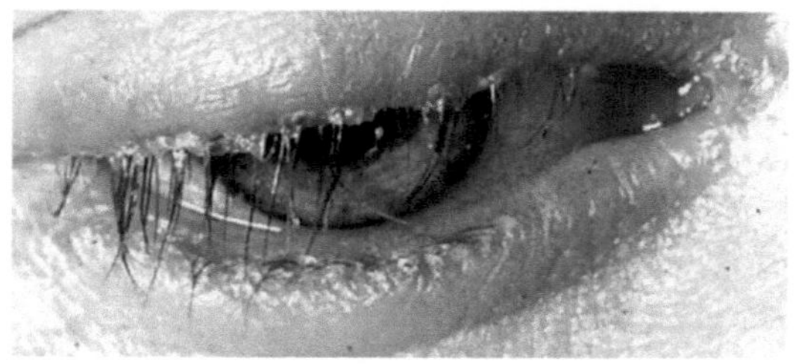

Blepharitis. Symptoms:

- Palpebral rim stinging
- Reddening of the palpebral rim and conjunctiva

Treatment:

- Hygiene
- Antibiotic Ointment

CONNATAL DISEASES

During the fertile age and during pregnancy it is necessary to make strict controls to the woman since acquiring some diseases such as rubella, chickenpox, cytomegalovirus, toxoplasmosis, herpes, syphilis, HIV, can cause visual impairment and blindness in the unborn child.

NEWBORN

Newborns should be evaluated in the first weeks of life to verify the transparency of the ocular media, called red reflex test, which can be normal or altered called leukocoria (white pupil), thus ruling out congenital cataracts and other corneal opacities that cause severe visual impairment and should be treated very early.

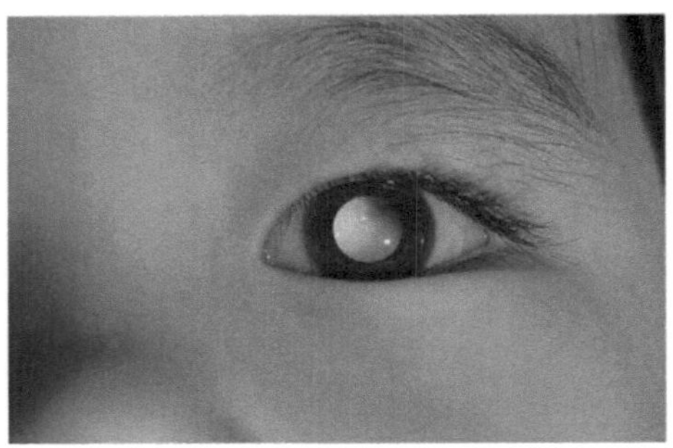

Leukocoria.

Conjunctivitis is very frequent in neonates, generally appearing between the 2nd and 5th day of life, its clinical picture is characterized by being uni or bilateral, with scarce to moderate mucopurulent secretion. It is generally self-limited and treatment is based on periodic hygiene.

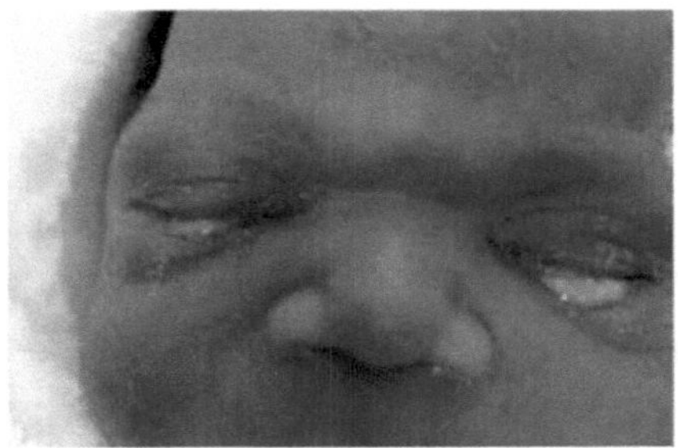

Neonatal conjunctivitis.

Always refer to an ophthalmologist. If the child was born prematurely and received oxygen therapy care, he/she may develop Retinopathy of prematurity (ROP), the leading cause of blindness in childhood, and should be closely monitored by a physician.

CONJUNTIVITIS

It is the inflammatory reaction of the conjunctiva. It may be of origin:

- Bacterial
- Viral
- Allergic

Signs and symptoms:

- Red eye
- Tearing
- Foreign body sensation
- Discharge, watery, mucopurulent or seromucous depending on the cause.
- Palpebral edema
- Pain

Treatment:

- Topical antibiotics: tobramycin, ciprofloxacin, erythromycin (in infants and pregnant women). 1 drop every 4 hours for at least 1 week.
- Indicate the correct hygiene of eyelids and eyelashes.
- Local cold

Important:

- Do not occlude these eyes as we favor microbial proliferation.
- Indicate isolation of the patient due to the risk of contagion.
- It is suggested never to indicate corticosteroids without a diagnosis of certainty due to the risk of generating herpetic activation.

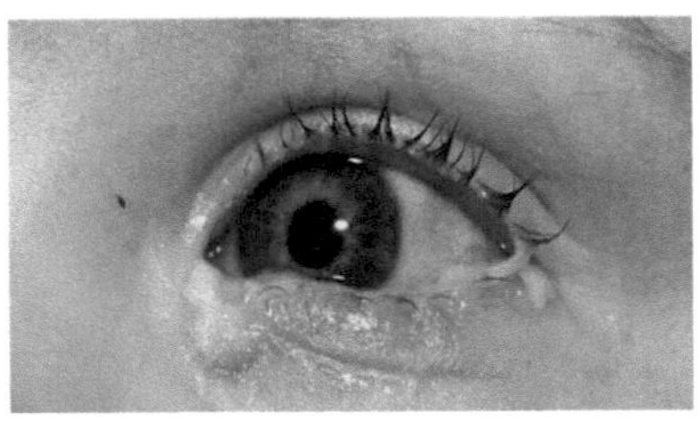

Conjunctivitis bacterial.

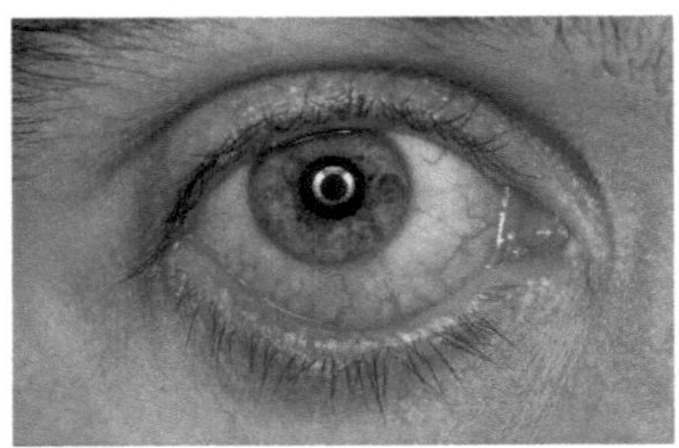

Viral conjunctivitis.

CHERATITIS

It is the inflammatory lesion of the corneal epithelium, stroma or both.

Signs and Symptoms:

- Red eye
- Foreign body sensation/pain/pain/ache
- Arenilla
- Photophobia
- Blurred vision.

Causes:

Bacteria, Viruses (Herpes), Fungi (Contact Lens Wearers), Traumatic (Contact Lens), Burns (Photoelectric, Welding), Dry Eye, Exposure (Facial Paralysis).

Treatment:

Topical lubricants - Topical antibiotics

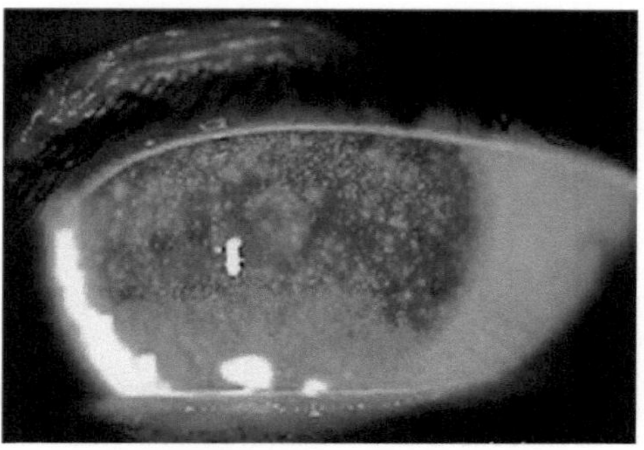

Keratitis sicca (per eye dry).

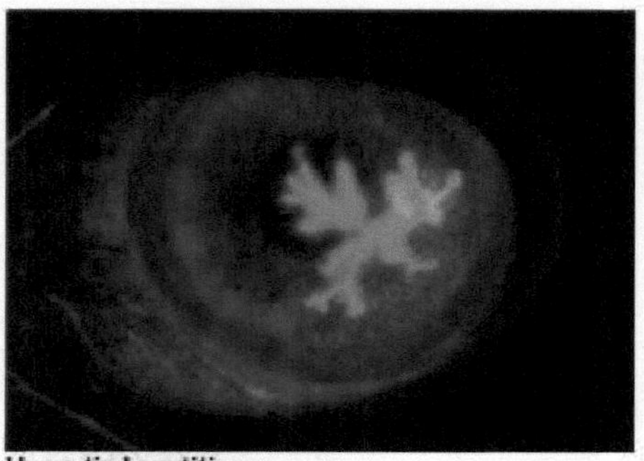

Herpetic keratitis.

SUBCONJUNCTIVAL HEMORRHAGE

It is the rupture of a capillary vessel in the space between the conjunctiva and the sclera. Hemorrhage is observed without signs of inflammation. Its evolution is spontaneous resolution in 1 to 2 weeks.

Signs and symptoms:

- Hemorrhagic subconjunctival stain
- Painless
- No inflammation
- Sudden onset

Causes:

HTA - Cough - Vomiting - Sudden exertion (without corticoids) 1 drop every 4 hours.

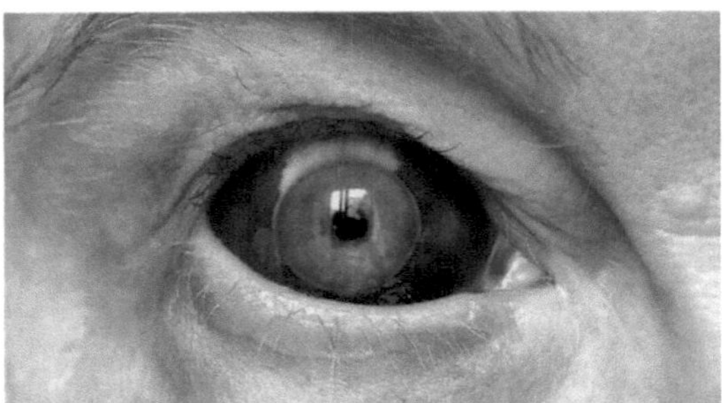

Subconjunctival hemorrhage.

STYE/CHALAZION

It is the infection of the palpebral moll, zeiss or meibomian glands, with the consequent development of a cyst with purulent material.

Symptoms:

- Localized swelling of the eyelid
- Pain
- Palpebral palpebral cyst

Treatment:

Topical antibiotic ointment: tobramycin, ciprofloxacin or erythromycin.

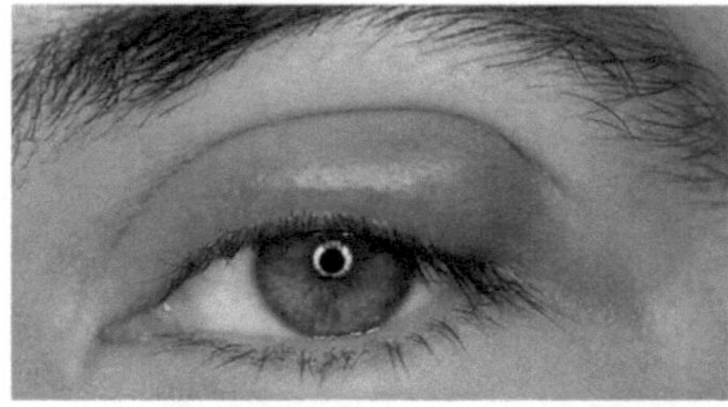

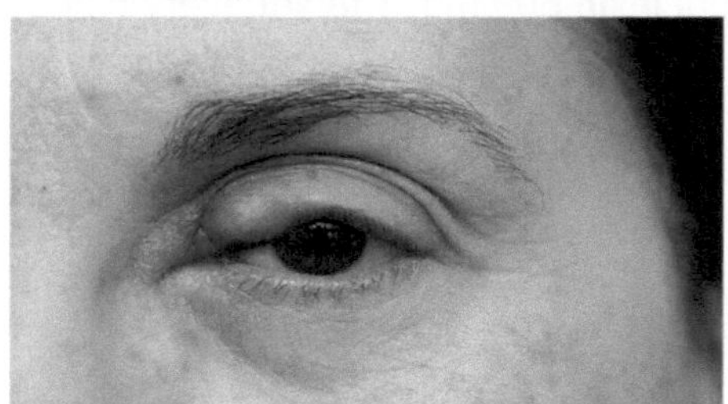

Stye. Chalazion.

PRESEPTAL CELLULITIS

It is the infection of the eyelid tissues anterior to the palpebral septum.

Symptoms:

- Sties/chalazion
- Insect bites
- Trauma

Signs and symptoms:

- Palpebral edema
- Palpebral swelling
- Preserved eye movements
- Localized pain
- Fever

Treatment:

Oral antibiotic, cephalexin 500 mg. 1 tablet every 6 hours. - Systemic anti-inflammatory drugs - Local cold

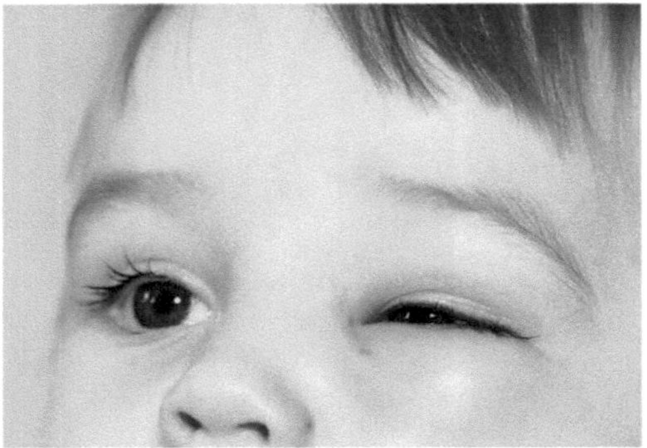

Preseptal cellulitis.

Orbital or Postseptal Cellulitis

It is the infection of the tissues of the orbit posterior to the palpebral septum. It is caused by dissemination of inflammatory/infectious processes of the paranasal sinuses or other tissues close to the orbit. The diagnosis is clinical. The condition is severe and may be complicated by cavernous sinus thrombosis.

Signs and symptoms:

- Palpebral edema
- Chemosis
- Fever
- General state commitment
- Pain
- Decreased vision
- Limitation of eye movements
- Diplopia
- Proptosis
- Compromised pupillary reflexes

Treatment: Hospitalization and intravenous antibiotics.

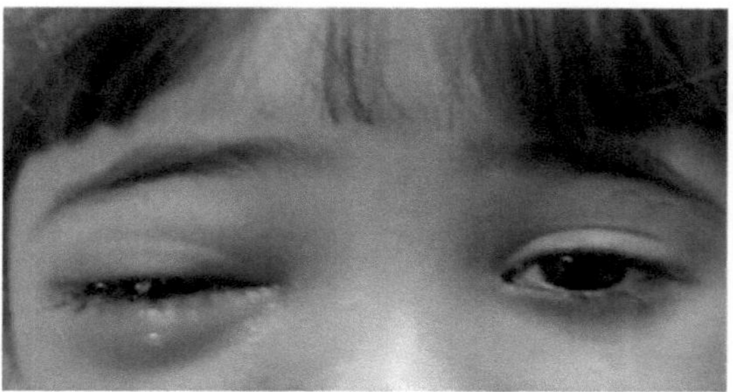

Obritory cellulitis.

HERPES ZOSTER OPHTHALMICUS

It is the involvement of the trigeminal territory by reactivation of the varicella zoster virus.

Signs and symptoms:

- Vesicles in the trigeminal territory
- Neuralgia
- Paresthesias
- Crusts

Treatment:

Acyclovir 800 mg. 5 times a day - Analgesics

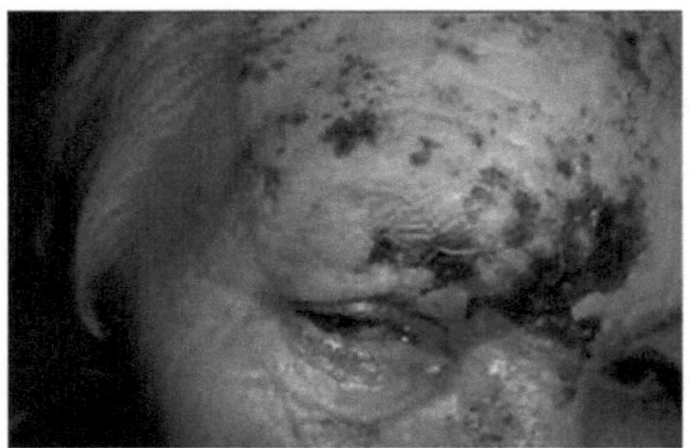

Herpes zoster ophthalmic.

Dacryocystitis

It is the inflammation of the obstructed lacrimal sac with superinfection of the lacrimal sac.

Signs and symptoms:

- Fever
- Localized pain
- Inflammation of the lacrimal sac

• Tearing

Treatment: Topical and systemic antibiotics (cephalexin) - Anti-inflammatory agents

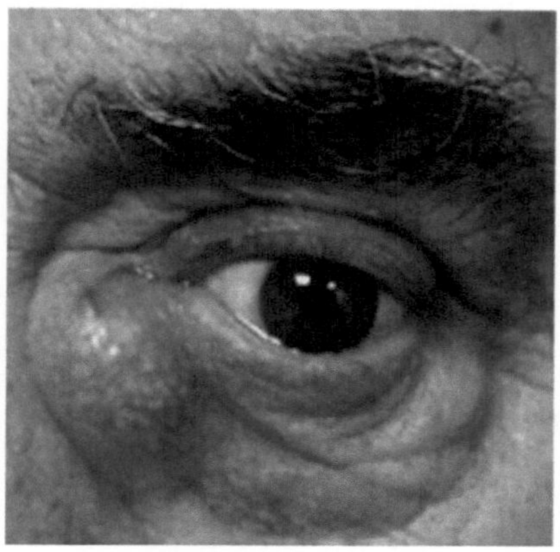

Dacryocystitis.

CHAPTER 4
OPHTHALMOLOGIC EMERGENCIES

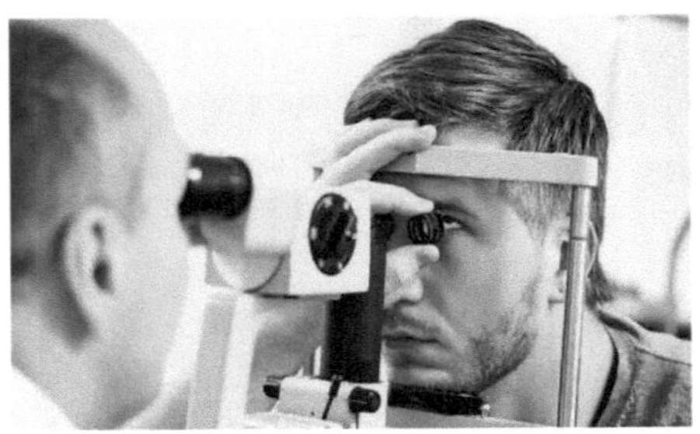

At this point we will define which are the urgent pathologies in order to identify them.

EMERGENCIES

The ophthalmologic emergencies are constituted by traumatisms, cuts, burns, caused by accidents, cuts, sand, glass or other accidents, punctures, presence of sand, glass or other foreign bodies in the eye. They should be referred immediately to the ophthalmologist or ophthalmological center more close. Among vision pathologies, only acute glaucoma requires urgent treatment.

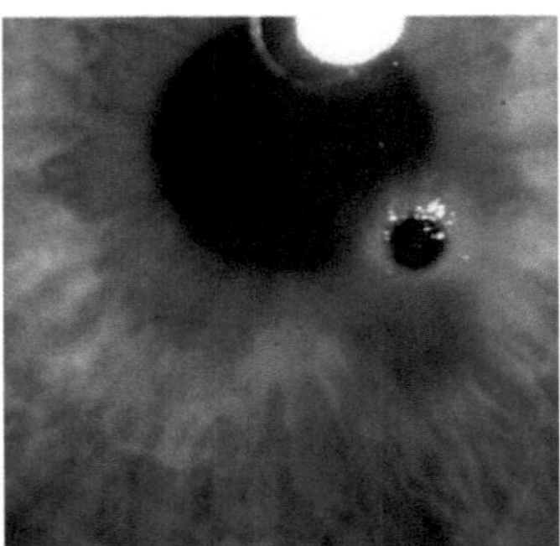

Metallic foreign body in cornea.

GLAUCOMA ACUTE

It is the sudden elevation of ocular pressure caused by blockage of the outflow of aqueous humor from the iridocorneal angle.

Signs and Symptoms:

- Severe eye pain
- Blurred and haloed vision around lights
- Cornea with loss of brightness
- Pupil in mid mydriasis
- Red and congestive eye (unilateral)
- May be accompanied by nausea
- Stony consistency of the eye when pressure is evaluated digitally (compare with contralateral eye).

Treatment:

Urgent referral to specialist

Important:

These episodes may be triggered by regular medication such as antispasmodics.

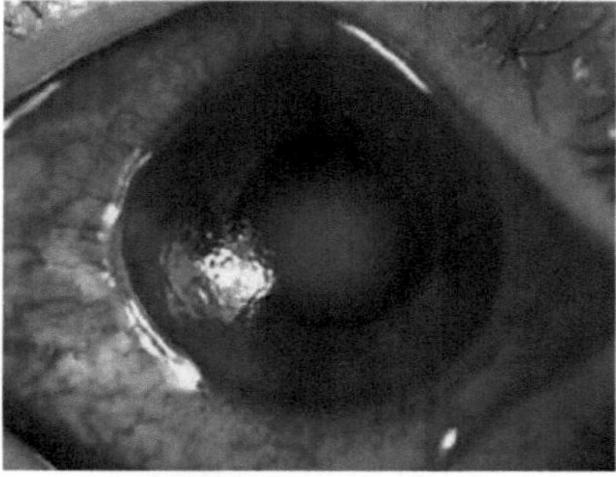

Acute glaucoma.

CORNEAL ULCER

It is a lesion of the corneal surface produced by a foreign body, mechanical trauma, severe dry eye, etc.

Signs and Symptoms:

- History of trauma or dry eye
- Intense pain
- Foreign body sensation
- Photophobia
- Red eye
- Unilateral

Treatment:

Antibiotic eye drops - Ocular lubricants

Important:

Rule out the presence of a corneal or subtarsal foreign body - In case of diagnostic doubt, do not occlude - Never prescribe anesthetics - Do not prescribe corticosteroids: they delay healing.

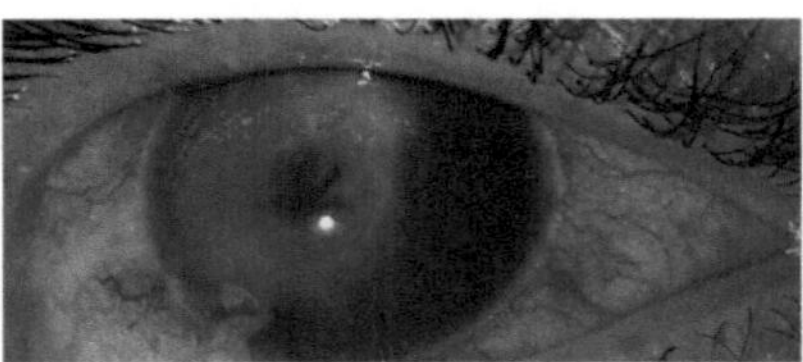

Corneal ulcer

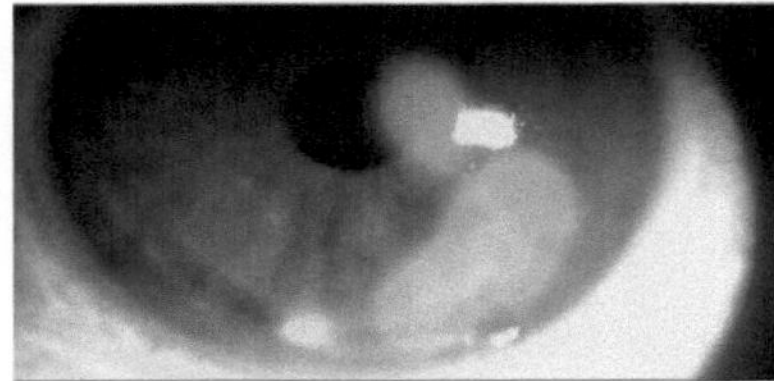

Tinted corneal ulcers with fuorescein.

Burns

Acid burns

The elements that most frequently generate this type of lesions are sulfuric acids or bacterial acids, hydrochloric acid, acetic acid, etc. These products generate coagulation of the corneal epithelium, which acts as a barrier to penetration that limits and localizes the lesion.

Treatment:

- Wash with abundant liquid.
- Topical antibiotics and lubricants.

Alkali burns

It is a lesion of the ocular structures produced by alkaline substances, which produce persistent and progressive damage to the tissues while the chemical agent remains in contact with the eye. It produces severe damage to the cornea and conjunctiva, and may require grafts.

Treatment:

- Apply topical anesthesia (propavacaine or lidocaine) and perform a thorough eye wash to remove all debris.
- Refer to specialist

Important:

- Do not occlude if you are not sure that the alkali residues have been completely removed.

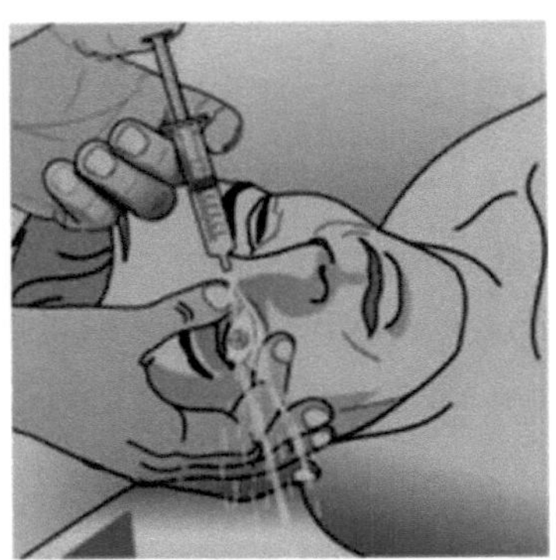

Post-burn eye wash.

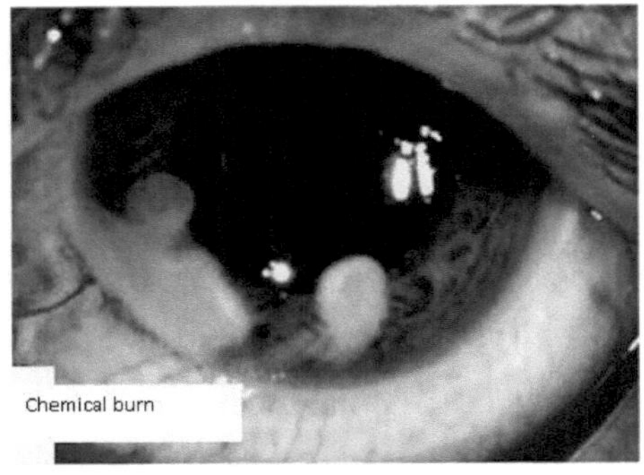

CHAPTER 5

WHEN TO DERIVE

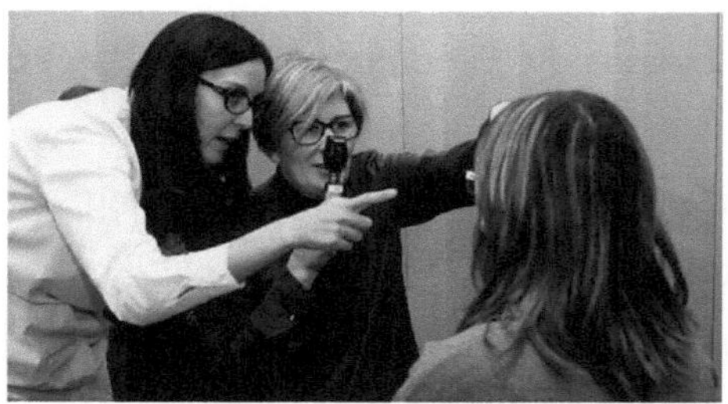

Refer all children (under 16 years of age inclusive), who have not had a check-up during the last year.

According to VISUAL ACCURACY

- Adult patient with VA less than 10/10 in one or both eyes
- Older adult patient, 40 years old, with near vision difficulty.

According to BACKGROUND

- Diabetic patient who has not had an eye exam in the last year.
- Hypertensive patient who has not had an eye exam in the last year.
- Patient with personal or family history of GLAUCOMA.
- Patient with acute ophthalmologic pathology at the time of examination in the last year.

OPHTHALMOLOGIC TRIAGE

The triage is a form with data on visual health that allows the control of the people visited by the health promoter and the health agent. Collect information regarding their visual health, family history, and visual acuity, as a guide for subsequent referral and determination, as well as statistical value.

BIBLIOGRAPHY

1) Newell F.: Ophthalmology, Fundamentals and Concepts, seventh edition, Mosby Publishing House, 1993 p. 257.

2) Deborah Pavan-Langston: Manual of Ocular Diagnosis and Therapy, fourth edition, Little, Brown and Company, 1996, pp. 117-118.

3) Kansky J.: Clinical Ophthalmology, second edition, Editorial Doyma, 1992, pp. 102-104.

4) The Wills Eye Manual, second edition, Lippincott Edit., 1994, p. 121-123.

5) Fraunfelder and Roy: Current Ocular Therapy, Saunders Ed., 1980, p. 571- 572.

6)Scheick-Leydhecker-Sampaolesi: Bases de la Oftalmología, eighteenth edition, Editorial Médica Panamericana, 1987, pp. 88-89.

7) Spalton D. - Hitchings R. - Hunter P.: Atlas of Clinical Ophthalmology, second edition, Editorial Mosby Doyma, 1995, pp. 5.21-.

8) Bruce E. Onofrey - Leonid Skorin, Jr. - Nicky R. Holdeman, Ocular Therapeutics Handbook -A Clinical Manual- Lippincott-Raven - Publishers. First edition. Pg. 74-75

9) Marinho Jorge Scarpa, Mauro Silveira de Quiroz Campos, Ana Luisa Hôfling de Lima: Conductas Terapêuticas em Oftalmologia; Editora Roca Ltda. 1999, p. 25.

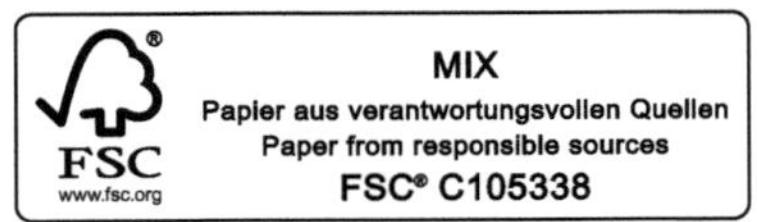

Printed by Books on Demand GmbH, Norderstedt / Germany